Parting

Published in

association with the

Foundation for End-of-Life Care

and the

P. L. Dodge Foundation

Parting

A HANDBOOK FOR SPIRITUAL CARE

NEAR THE END OF LIFE

JENNIFER SUTTON HOLDER &

JANN ALDREDGE-CLANTON

The University of North Carolina Press

Chapel Hill and London

Library of Congress
Cataloging-in-Publication Data

Holder, Jennifer Sutton.

Parting: a handbook for spiritual care near
the end of life / Jennifer Sutton Holder and
Jann Aldredge-Clanton.

  p. cm.

ISBN 978-0-8078-5529-4 (pbk.: alk. paper)

1. Death. 2. Spiritual life. I. Aldredge-Clanton,
Jann, 1946– II. Title.

BD444.H58   2004

155.9′37—DC22   2003021553

12 11 10 09 08   6 5 4 3 2

Contents

Foreword

This handbook seeks specifically to assist anyone who chooses to serve as a close companion for a terminally ill relative or friend. These companions are truly the unsung heroes of end-of-life care. Our hope is that the handbook will teach them how to include spiritual care in companionship.

What do we mean by spiritual care? Spiritual care for the purpose of this handbook is soul care, helping the human spirit in its search for peace. It is the attempt to help those near the end of life feel whole, fulfilled, and in harmony with their world and their higher power. Religious experience may or may not be spiritual, and spiritual experience may or may not be religious. Regardless of the dying person's religious persuasion or faith tradition, spiritual care near the end of life supplies a deep human need.

The handbook is the result of many months of vision, inspiration, dedication, and hard work. It reflects insights gained from numerous interviews with persons who have accompanied others at the end of life: hospice professionals, nurses, physicians, and other health care–givers; ministers of many faiths; friends and family. We also interviewed men and women as they approached death. From a rabbi, to a priest, to a Muslim imam, to a native American spiritual leader, to a practitioner of Christian Science, and to many others we went, researching this handbook.

The time leading up to conducting the interviews was

consumed by conversations between Dr. Larry Churchill and me. We were joined later by Rev. Luther Jones. These conversations focused upon our deep concerns that there were large numbers of people dying every day with unmet spiritual needs, and that it was their closest companions who seemed to be in the best position to meet those needs. During this period the vision for the handbook crystallized, along with a plan to use interviews as the basis for its content.

In an effort to identify the ideal authors, I sought guidance from Travis Maxwell, whom I remembered as chaplain on the oncology unit at Baylor University Medical Center in Dallas when I practiced there in the 1970s and 1980s. Travis delivered pastoral care and spiritual care to critically ill patients and families with effectiveness and skill, a highly valued member of the caregiving team on the unit. It was Travis who led us to the handbook's authors, Jennifer Sutton Holder and Jann Aldredge-Clanton. I want to express my sincere appreciation to them and to all of those persons along the way who, through numerous excited conversations, gave inspiration and encouragement to this effort.

It is not my intention to dedicate this work to any specific person or persons, other than those countless personal companions who have taken care of a terminally ill relative or friend, especially those who have encountered and addressed an unmet spiritual need in the final journey of life. I would, however, like to mention my mother, Annie Laurie Beckham Williams, and mother-in-law, Rosalind Repp Jennings, both of whom served with compassion and skill as spiritual companions for their husbands.

> J. Richard Williams, M.D., *Chairman and President*
> *Foundation for End-of-Life Care*

Acknowledgments

The authors would like to thank the following individuals who offered their time and insight during interviews for this book: Rev. Joe Davis; Rev. Thom McLeod; Rev. Harold Wallace; Esther Colliflower, R.N.; Sarah McKinnon, M.A.; Rev. Luther Jones; Rev. Hugh Westbrook; Rev. Kelvin Calloway; Rev. Travis Maxwell; Barry Kinzbrunner, M.D.; Rev. Martha Rutland; Robert Fine, M.D.; Rev. Joseph Driscoll; Christina Puchalski, M.D.; Rev. Mica Togami; Richard Payne, M.D.; Gwen London, Ph.D.; Rev. Sol Bird Mockisin; Rev. Ella McCarroll; Rev. Betty Clark; Rev. Richard B. Fife; Kathleen Foley, M.D.; Dr. Lobsang Rapgay; Giulia Plum; Jean Jolly, Ph.D.; Rabbi Simkha Weintraub; Rev. Don Smidt; Marcia Guntzel Feldman; Imam Yusuf Hasan; Rev. Francis Rivers Mesa; Rev. Karen Black; Rev. R. Mark Grace; J. R. Williams, M.D.; and Wendy Deering-Poynter.

The authors thank Rev. Bob Duncan, Ph.D., and Rev. Mike Mullender, Ph.D., for their assistance in conducting interviews. We also thank Howard W. Stone, Ph.D., and Karen M. Stone as primary editors and contributors. Rev. Luther Jones; Larry Churchill, Ph.D.; and J. R. Williams, M.D., also helped in editing the manuscript, and we thank Sandy Grotegeer for providing valuable technical assistance.

Introduction

Why are we here?
How can we understand and find meaning in suffering?
What is death, and what happens after death?

To ask and seek answers to these questions is to engage in spiritual work. This volume is a handbook on spiritual care of the dying, yet its purpose is not to address these big questions per se—still less to answer them. Rather, it serves as a practical guide to how people who are dying tend to approach these questions and how their friends and family may act as companions to accompany them on this final journey.

The authors, as hospital chaplains, have themselves provided this companionship to the dying many times and have also witnessed it in others. They recognize the need to offer people some simple advice that can bring peace during a time of great emotion, upheaval, and change. They are skilled and trustworthy guides to the spiritual work of the dying and to those who seek to provide compassionate convoy at life's end.

It's worth taking a moment here to consider what "spiritual work" might mean to different readers. Until fairly recently, spirituality as a type of experience separate from a particular religious tradition was an unfamiliar notion. That is no longer the case; in contemporary American society, discussions about spirituality sometimes have little or nothing to do with organized religion. So a few definitions relevant to this book may be helpful.

By "religion" most people mean an institution with certain beliefs and rituals and a history shared by a community of observant or faithful members. To identify oneself as religious ordinarily implies that one is an observant Jew, Buddhist, Muslim, Christian, Hindu, and so on. In contrast, "spirituality" has come to mean a more individualized and personal engagement with whatever is sacred or transcendent in life. This perspective may or may not involve religion. Nor does it necessarily involve convictions about a spirit world or an image of human beings as consisting of bodies and spirits. Rather "spirituality" usually signals a belief that there is more to life than what is evident on the surface, a deeper meaning to human existence than the accumulation of material fortune and fame, and a recognition of the profound meaning in human relationships. Spirituality often signals a broad search for ultimate meaning in life and an appreciation of the many different ways people can affirm a transcendent dimension.

In this book, "spirituality" should be thought of in the most inclusive sense. For many readers, it will simply refer to the religious faith with which they are affiliated. For others, it will mean an individual and personal sense of what is ultimate or sacred in their lives. This book embraces the widest possible range of meanings of the "spiritual" without subscribing to any particular beliefs or practices. In this sense spirituality is a common human activity, an activity of seeking deeper meaning in oneself, in relationships, and in life. Eventually, every person's spiritual search will include a need for spiritual care, as he or she confronts the meaning of life's end and the ultimate loss of death.

From its inception, this volume has been thought of as a handbook. There is a long tradition of handbooks, both in spiritual work and in other fields, including such things as daily meditations and pocket guides on everything from fly fishing to table etiquette. Our goal was to produce a guide to spiritual companionship that would, like other handbooks, be handy and portable, something that could be slipped into a pocket or purse, something that could be read or reread quickly, and something to which thoughtful readers could contribute based on their own experiences. If this volume is widely used and shared, carried into homes, hospitals, or places of worship, and even revised based on the experiences of our readers, we will have achieved our goal.

Larry R. Churchill, Ph.D.
Ann Geddes Stahlman Professor of Medical Ethics
Vanderbilt University

1 Setting Out

Doug was an active, happy man spending his retirement years instructing others in golf. For a time, he brushed off the nagging pain in his lower back, thinking he had wrenched his muscles with a golf swing. But the pain intensified, and Doug learned that he had a malignant tumor on his spine. From a full life, he abruptly entered the process of dying. It took only a few weeks for him to die.

During that brief time, Doug chose to enter an inpatient hospice (a facility and program that is wholly devoted to helping people die in comfort and with dignity). He also immersed himself and his feelings in another of his lifelong pleasures: art. Doug's family brought him art supplies, admired his work, and even attached a little penlight to a baseball cap so that he could sketch through sleepless nights without disturbing others on his hospice ward. They collected his artworks, framed and displayed them near his bed, and listened as he told them about his drawings.

Doug wrote in his journal almost daily about the care of his nurses, the camaraderie with his doctors, and the visits from family members. His niece gave him a foot massage and pedicure when she came to visit. His sister reminisced and laughed with him about times past. He voiced his worries about his adult son and asked his sister to look after him. As he grew weaker, his sketches became less detailed. Then, as his life drew to a close, the sketches were only a few stark lines, the journal entries a few words.

Doug's dying wasn't all creativity and companionship. He suffered terrible pain, dark days when he felt despondent, restless nights he thought would never end. But, surrounded with his artworks and people he loved, he died with his work finished, with dignity and acceptance.

What would we give to have such peace surround the death of one we love? Of course, sometimes it is out of our reach. We have no control over sudden death, for example, and mean-spirited relatives can make a person's last days and hours more difficult than they ought to be. The dying may suffer from dementia and be unable to converse or even recognize family members. But it is possible, more often than people think, for death to be a spiritual blessing to those who are leaving as well as those who are left behind. Peace and meaning can light the way.

Offering Spiritual Companionship

When you sign on to be a spiritual companion, you enter a two-way street. You invite intimacy, and you share from your own soul. You are a source of strength, but you look to the dying person for inspiration and moments of strength as well.

You open the window for peace to surround the one who is dying, and you feel its breeze on your face.

You look for truth, for the expression of candid and deep feelings ranging from agony and anger to joy and acceptance, and find you must bare your feelings also.

Both of you will grow. You will care for one another. And

you both will find tears to be a healing release and closeness of body, mind, and spirit to be a shelter from the cold night of pain and grief.

The journey of spiritual companionship at the end of life begins *now*. Set out on the path today, while there are still time and energy to devote to the road ahead. The person who receives a life-threatening diagnosis needs your spiritual companionship from the first moment onward.

One physician says that the best way to improve spiritual care for the dying is to improve it for the living. All too often, the day-to-day business of life gets in the way of the inner life. Death clears the calendar; it uncrowds life so that spiritual needs come to the forefront. It is painful to face mortality alone, and most persons who are dying will welcome your support and presence.

If distance separates you from your loved one who is going to die, and you will not be able to travel both now and later, seriously consider going *now*. You can have a memorial service later, in your own hometown, but you will never regret the time you spend with this loved one who is still alive, still breathing, thinking, loving, questioning, finding a way.

Itineraries: Stops on Spiritual Journeys

Where might a spiritual journey take you and your companion? What is the destination you seek together? Is this a journey you even want to contemplate taking?

Death calls forth the most intense of human emotions, both for the one who is dying and for the spiritual companion. It compels the travelers to search out every spiritual tool they have ever collected, to cry out to their higher power for help, to tap into every coping mechanism and source of strength they have ever used before. Death often presents nothing short of a spiritual crisis, both for the one who is dying and for the companion. The very act of admitting that death is the unavoidable destination of the journey requires facing an acutely painful reality.

The spiritual "dis-ease" of either the companion or the one who is dying can pose obstacles to spiritual companionship. Both travelers must rely primarily on their current level of spiritual maturity and familiar spiritual resources. The journey offers an unparalleled opportunity to expand their spiritual awareness and resources by trying new spiritual pathways together and consciously seeking spiritual adventure and awakenings. They will undoubtedly encounter rough spiritual terrain, and their road must go *through* these hard and painful places, not around.

What are some of the stops along the way they might anticipate on this spiritual journey? Their itinerary might include the following "spiritual moments":

Wholeness: The sense of being complete in oneself.
A sense of basic inner integrity. Said one spiritual pilgrim, "I felt as though the battle had finally stopped. Floating there on the water I lacked nothing, thirsted for nothing, was dissatisfied with nothing about myself. It was a moment of absolute calm, a sense of profound fulfillment."

Belonging: The feeling of being at home, or at the proper place in time. A sense of participation in one's world, of connectedness to others and to one's environment.

Gratitude: An awareness of and receptivity toward the gifts that enrich one's life. Recognition of the presence of resources, experiences, relationships, and objects that have no connection to one's efforts. In a moment of gratitude, one spiritual wayfarer said, "My favorite thing is watching the sun rise on the bay in the morning. Sometimes I just sit there and say 'Thank you, God.' It's a beautiful gift."

Humility: The ability to love oneself in spite of oneself. Acceptance of limitations, awareness of capacities, respect for the mysterious aspects of oneself all are part of humility. One man reflected, "I'm a pretty average painter. But when I'm painting I don't have to think about how I measure up. And every now and then, something happens . . . and I surprise myself."

Reverence: A sense of wonder and awe; of vastness, greatness, complexity; of being taken outside of oneself.

Perspective: Seeing deeply into things. An intuitive awareness of meanings. Insight or wisdom about oneself or one's life situation.

Trust: Moving into and with the current of an experience or a relationship. Surrendering control of outcomes and conditions. Depending on persons or forces outside the range of one's immediate control. One person said, "You really have to believe that people aren't going to let you go. . . . I was shaking and crying. But for one time I was able to trust somebody else."

Devotion: Commitment to care for someone/something. Experiencing the other (or an aspect of oneself) as a valued part of one's life. Devotion came to one man in the form of a dog: "I got her (a golden retriever) because through all these years of drugging—living

out of cars, in the gutter, stealing, selling, all that —
I never had one thing I took care of, except my habit.
It's a start about being loyal to or responsible for
something."

Release: The experience of being liberated, unburdened,
or rescued from compulsive drives or anxieties.
"I begin . . . with all kinds of worries, stress, or
frustration. And most of the time it just feels like
I literally outrun them. . . . They are far behind me.
I feel lighter."

These are only a few of the stops along the way of a journey of spiritual companionship. Your stops will be as individual as your itinerary, as interesting and replenishing as you make them.

Two Levels of Needs: Physical and Spiritual

Two issues loom large at the end of life: managing pain and having spiritual needs met. The medical team—doctors, nurses, and hospice and other caregivers—certainly will do what they can to ease pain with medical and physical means. There is much you can do as well. This handbook will suggest some simple methods that will help with your loved one's physical comfort. But professional end-of-life caregivers also have learned that attending to spiritual needs often brings relief from pain, or improves ability to cope with it.

As Manuel lay dying, he expressed deep anguish over years of alienation from Tony, his son. Manuel's pain had become unmanageable, and regrets tormented him. A sister managed to track Tony down. She found him eager to end the isolation from his father, but his situation made it impossible to come immediately. In the meantime Tony tape-recorded a message to his father, telling him that he loved him and wanted to let the past go. When Manuel heard the tape, he wept. Then he listened to it again and again. As it played, his pain diminished, and so Manuel found both physical and spiritual comfort from his son's words of reconciliation.

Body and soul are, we think, inseparable. Spiritual care is every bit as important as physical care at the end of life. You offer a gift to even consider spiritual companionship for the one who is dying. The voices of past experience assure you that gifts await you, as well. Let's begin!

2 A Personal Journey

Emmy lived in Miami, Florida. She had battled cancer for two years, and she knew she was dying. Above all, Emmy wanted to die at home. But this was 1978, and no hospices existed in southern Florida. Emmy heard of some visionary people who were trying to begin a program of comfort care for the dying, and she offered to be their guinea pig. "I know you don't know what you're doing. But if you help me die at home, I'll teach you how to do it," she told them.

Emmy's personal journey toward death became a mission. She bared her body and her soul to those who came to accompany her. Some days were good days. Other days, she said the kindest thing would be to shoot her. Emmy's life had always been devoted to causes, and her final cause was to teach a fledgling hospice team—and her own family—how to be her spiritual companions as she died, at home, on her own terms.

Companions Welcome

Emmy's story illustrates how very personal the journey toward death is for each one of us. The unique blend of culture, family history, religious tradition, personality, and physical and spiritual characteristics that make people who they are in life also shape who they will be in death. The one who is dying must lead the way.

Few people want their departure from life to be solitary. Isolation and loneliness are unutterably painful at the end of life, and terminally ill people usually treasure companionship of any sort. Emmy loved to have people come in and read the day's headlines, watch the news on television, and tell her about their day.

For other dying people, the sounds of grandchildren playing nearby, pots clanking in the kitchen, or the coming and going of family and nurses and aides keep them in the circle of life. Often, when their condition requires a hospital bed, hospice patients request that it be placed in the middle of the living room or den, not back in the bedroom. They want to be a part of the family until the very end. Of course, they may occasionally request that a door be closed for privacy, or that there be quiet so they can rest.

Just as people who provide clinical care for the dying must bring medical instruments and supplies, spiritual companions need to pack specialized gear for spiritual conversations. A number of hospice workers and veteran travelers with the dying have suggested tools to help the family and close friends who wish to become spiritual travelers with loved ones nearing the end of life.

Packing for the Road Ahead

As you prepare for this important journey, you will not need to go to school for advanced training or visit a shopping mall to acquire exotic tools. You will be packing from your own spiritual inventory. You need to know where you are on your own spiritual path, and seek strength from your higher power.

Keep in the front of your mind—and this will be repeated throughout the handbook—that you are a companion, not a leader. You will not have to make this trip alone. You are not responsible for the outcome. You have no control over the timing.

It is better to think of the list that follows, and other lists in this handbook, as a menu of choices rather than a checklist. You may find only one or two of these suggestions to be helpful in your situation. Choose only what seems comfortable and natural for you and for your loved one, and discard the rest. If any of this starts to feel like a chore, you probably are trying too hard.

PRESENCE

The simple fact that you are willing to be there is a gift. Your stated or unstated promise, "I will come back; I will not abandon you," is probably the most important message of spiritual care. Our mere presence communicates to the dying that they are not alone, that we will be with them to the end.

LISTENING

Dying persons are dealing with ultimate questions about the meaning of life. They don't need your answers or solutions—just your listening ears.

Your body language communicates that you are listening.

Sit by the bedside. Look into the person's eyes. This is a time when the dying person should definitely be in charge, a time to express thoughts and wishes freely without advice or pressure to believe or feel differently.

ACCEPTANCE

Accept the reality that death is near, as difficult as that may be. After that, affirm that this person's life and achievements have meaning. Ask, "What do you value now? What do you define as quality of life at this point?" Offer assurance of value and love. Keep in mind that acceptance also means honestly talking about past actions that may have caused hurt or anger in others.

Setting aside your own agenda will help you and the dying person. In fact, the presence, conversation, and support you give to this loved one will help you immensely in your own grief work, both now and in the future.

CANDOR

Make it clear that your dying companion can talk to you about anything—what no one else wants to hear, or what no one else should hear. It may be necessary to clear the air about the person's guilt and resentment over long-ago hurt feelings, misunderstandings, or misdeeds. Whether or not these issues from the past can ever be resolved, there is sometimes healing just in the telling.

You may also find it important to discuss what your loved one does or does not want done in the event of a crisis that requires a ventilator or a feeding tube, additional treatments, or medical procedures. Such conversations about physical subjects often have an intensely spiritual quality. Expression of last wishes can bring comfort at the end of life by restoring one's power, freedom, and sense of control.

PATIENCE

You may already have discovered the need for patience in the first hours after an accident, heart attack, stroke, or other health catastrophe.

Carrie described her first quarter hour with her mother in the intensive care unit (ICU) as extremely uncomfortable. She didn't know what to do. Here lay the foundation of the family, beautiful hair shaved off, left side of her face slack, gardener's tan turned yellowish, shunts and respirators and tubes attached at every angle. Carrie thought, "I need time to get used to this." She sat silently by the bedside, gazing steadily at her mother's face until she felt more at ease, then began a conversation full of tears and touching, blessings and songs, that will go with her for the rest of her life.

Be prepared to tolerate mood changes and mixed feelings, both in yourself and in the one who is dying. For example, a young mother, terminally ill with cancer, said she felt like she was on a roller coaster—at the top praying for a miracle so that she could see her daughter grow up, but at the lowest point crying, "God, please take me away."

Even the upper end of a mood swing can be disconcerting for the spiritual companion. Already beginning to grieve the loss of your loved one, you walk in the room one morning and find a chirpy, joke-cracking dynamo in place of the tearful, pain-wracked person you kissed good night twelve hours earlier. It throws you off balance.

You may find it helpful to begin each new watch somewhat tentatively and quietly, taking time to sense your dear one's condition and mood, and adjusting your responses accordingly. A few quiet breaths, a silent prayer, or some mental instructions to yourself (as Carrie used to get her initial discomfort under control) may help you stay afloat on rapidly changing physical and emotional tides.

Patience also means becoming comfortable with silence. This is a time to listen quietly. It is a time to hear messages in unspoken words, in what is not said as well as what is said. Pauses can be as important as dialogue. This is not a time to attempt to persuade your loved one into assuming your way of thought, perception, or belief.

Indeed, patience and a silent presence may be the best spiritual gift you can offer. The saying "Don't just stand there; do something!" needs reversing here: "Don't just do something; sit there!"

ADVOCACY

Let your loved one tell you, "I'd like you to take care of me this way" and describe his or her wishes to you in detail. This enables you to leave out what is not important and focus on what is. Almost certainly you will need to be an advocate for the wishes of the person nearing the end of life. You may be asked to help prepare a will or living will. You may have more knowledge of all the available choices, and you have more strength to research options. If these practical issues are not addressed, they can block the path to spiritual peace.

As spiritual companion, you will also be a care manager to help achieve the greatest comfort level, whether that means seeking a hospice referral, requesting more adequate pain medication, or removing unwanted nutrition. Another gift of spiritual companionship is to understand that, when the soul is about to take flight, the body no longer needs or desires food. You can stop pushing food and water on a patient who no longer desires it or who even becomes nauseous after eating or drinking. The absence of nutrients and fluids is nature's way of bringing gentle closure and even pain relief as the body gradually shuts down. Just using a small sponge or swab or tiny shavings of ice to give a drop or two of moisture can be the kindest nourishment to a dying person.

Being an advocate may mean shedding some of your natural inclinations or preconceived notions. The comfort of the one who is dying comes first.

Dying can be so deadly serious. Spiritual care calls for time to laugh. Both the patient and the companion need relief from the heavy burden they carry toward a destination they may dread. There are humorous moments to enjoy along the way. One hospice patient had been burdened for years with the high cost of his prescription medications. On hearing that the hospice would provide his drugs at no cost, he quipped, "Well, then, let's load up!"

Velma had requested that all life support, including nutrition and water, be removed so she could die. As aides transferred her to a bed in the comfort care section, her leg pain made the job more difficult. Velma quipped, "Well, I guess I should be doing my exercises!" Her family laughed, cried, and marveled that, of all of them, it was she who could lighten up the sorrowful atmosphere with a little joke.

Whenever you can, enjoy what is humorous about the situations you encounter.

COURAGE

It takes courage to face bad news. It takes courage to risk feeling vulnerable with one another. It takes courage to face the hard questions: Why me? Why now? Did I do something wrong? Is this my fault?

You can say, "I am not afraid to face this with you," or, "I am afraid, but we can face this together." You summon up courage to stay with and validate all the feelings of the one who is dying, whatever those feelings are—fear, anger, pain, guilt, joy, or peace.

DEPENDABILITY

Do what you say you are going to do. If you promise to come for a visit tomorrow at four, come tomorrow at four. No matter what is going on in your life, come.

Don't shy away from rough days. Don't think your loved one will not want you there because she or he is in intense pain. To provide spiritual care, go wherever the journey leads. By your actions, offer this deeply comforting message: "I want to do this with you, and I will be there, no matter what."

HOPE

Bring a suitcase full of hope along with you.

Change the focus of hope to what is achievable: hope for a day that is more comfortable, a day that affords a short conversation with a spouse or loved one, a day when a grandchild comes, a day when soup tastes good, a day to sit outside for a bit, a day when a hummingbird finds the feeder outside the window, a day to feel forgiveness or offer it.

Hope can be a traveling companion for both of you, if you give it new meanings.

CREATIVITY

At one hospice in England, the residents were brought into the sunny living room with a television set centered among them. The much-loved Wimbledon tennis classics were under way. Refreshments were tiny cups of raspberries and whipped cream. The spiritual journey begs for such creative moments when the ordinary becomes extraordinary because of some inspiration on the part of the dying person or the companion.

Creativity has no bounds, and in this crisis you may find that you are more creative than you ever thought possible. You might want to decorate your loved one's room for a special occasion (or no occasion at all). Bring in nicely matted artworks by children or grandchildren. Frame a poster of motorcycles, a particular artist, vintage radios, flowers, railroads—whatever the appropriate special interests. Invite a local jazz combo or a string quartet (or country and western gospel singers) to come to the room and perform.

Surprise is on your side as you exercise your creativity, but do keep in mind the tastes and personality of the one you are caring for. An old cynic is unlikely to be moved—and may even be disgusted—by balloons, cute floral arrangements, scented candles, or cheerful music.

SENSITIVITY

There are times for having spiritual conversations, and times for not even attempting them. On a day filled with dreadful pain, nausea, or fatigue, or when the bed linens are wet or soiled, explicitly spiritual conversations may find little place.

Being a spiritual companion means talking at opportune times and refraining from conversation at inopportune times. It means being sensitive to the dying person's daily mood, condition, and interest in talking about deeper things.

You may be caring for one who is afraid of emotions, runs from them, would rather die than express inner feelings. This is not the time to press new behavior ("Tell me your deepest feelings") on a crusty or taciturn relative. Spiritual content can be drawn from the well of comfortable, every-day talk — old times, sports, the weather, grandchildren, reci-pes — and especially from your own silent, steady presence.

CURIOSITY

The exploration of spiritual territory requires curiosity. Truly wanting to know more about the person nearing the end of life, whose likes and dislikes, wishes, personality, and beliefs are paramount, is a requisite for the traveling companion.

The dying, too, can continue to be curious, questioning, and open to new insights. One woman took pleasure in hearing new hymns, especially one from South Africa. She learned new prayers and used them in her meditations. How inspiring still to be growing spiritually on one's deathbed!

You will want to stay open to spiritual exploration with-out looking for particular right or wrong answers. Your loved one may have questions as well as profound reflec-tions on spiritual or theological themes, and you also should not be afraid to introduce new ideas or questions into the conversation just as long as you refrain from preaching or persuading.

TIME

This journey takes time and energy. Sometimes it seems to go on forever. Gaps between meaningful spiritual conversa-tions are long. Strength ebbs, and talk comes slowly. The spiritual companion needs to have (or take) time to be with the one who is dying. Time is needed to talk, to explore, to come to new awareness, and even to change one's think-ing now and then. When weary, remember this is the only time you will have to deepen your relationship and harvest friendship with this person.

Crossing the Bridge

If you have some of these things packed, you are well prepared for your journey alongside your loved one near the end of life. But sometimes you will find it hard to cross over from the superficial to the spiritual. It is like two people walking on either side of a rushing river. The noise of the water limits their conversation to simple interchanges across the way: "Hello!" "Where are you going?" "Nice day!"

COMING CLOSER

It is easy to let such a river flow between the one who is nearing death and the companion, but it is a river that limits conversation to the business of the day: "How are you today?" "What did the doctor say?" "What have you been able to eat?"

You need a bridge to cross the noisy river, to get closer to the person you care for, to be able to converse and hear each other plainly. The longer you walk side by side, the easier it will be for the conversations to grow more personal. Each of you can feel safe taking the lead on difficult topics once the bridge is crossed; each of you can trust the other.

SPIRITUAL CONVERSATION STARTERS

How do you cross the bridge? Certain starters have helped others to narrow the conversation gap. You may wish to ask the person near the end of life questions such as these, or to come up with your own questions.

If you don't mind telling me, I'd like to know what it's like to be you right now.

Is there anything you have wanted to tell me?

Where do you find your strength? Are there memories, inspirational passages, songs, or thoughts that keep you going?

What do you think about when you first wake up in the morning?

If your higher power were here, what would you say? What would you ask for?

How are other members of your family acting toward you now? How are they acting toward each other?

Would you like us to pray together? We can pray for each other silently, or one of us can start and the other can finish. Or I can pray for us both.

What is your greatest hope [fear, wish, etc.] right now?

If you and your loved one have not made a habit of discussing spiritual things in the past, you may find that it works better to take the initiative in sharing, leaving the dying person a place to respond. For example, you may wish to open a conversation with something along these lines.

Do you remember when _____?

I have always loved it when _____.

I am angry [or happy, or sad] about _____.

I hope for _____ right now; what are you hoping for?

I need to tell you several things: _____ [making sure you are not "dumping" too much of your own baggage on the one who is dying].

This time is scary for me; I don't know how you are feeling about it. I have some concerns—I would like to talk about them and hear how you feel about them, because I have no way of knowing.

I felt a divine presence with us when _____. Have you felt that presence lately? All these years we have never talked about _____.

I wonder what I would want to be remembered for. I think it would be _____. How about you?

I'm wondering what life will be like without you. These are the things I'll miss: _____. What will you miss? What do you most hate to leave behind?

If the person still resists talking about deeper things, don't push. You are not the one who is dying; you are just here for the companionship. You have other gifts to offer, such as presence, touch, music, and laughter.

Susan loved her father intensely, yet in his dying she couldn't seem to move the conversation past the daily "numbers game"—blood sugar, weight, pulse, oxygen level, outside temperature. She wanted to tell him how she loved him, how she would miss him, what a wonderful father he had been. But they skimmed the surface of each day until, on a return flight from a business trip, she made a list: "Your 10 Best Gifts." Then Susan waited for the right time. It came on a Sunday morning in her father's hospice room, when a television sermon addressed the need to balance life between work and family. Shyly, quietly, she said at the sermon's end, "Daddy, you always did that well. I was thinking on my way home about all the things you did well. I wrote down a list of your 10 best gifts to me. Want to hear them?" She read the list, and they cried. From then on, their conversations were not restricted to numbers but also went to deeper, richer places of the soul. Her father is gone now, but Susan keeps the list in her daily organizer and has the joy of knowing he heard exactly how she felt about him.

You will find your own bridge. Once you cross it, your loved one's final journey can become a blessing for both of you, an enriching and life-changing adventure.

3 Spiritual Scenery

Kate was terminally ill. She and her husband, Russell, under-stood that their time together would be short. Their evening ritual was to have a drink together. He would ring the bell and call out, "Post time!" She would have an orange juice, and he would drink scotch on the rocks. He always positioned the bed so they could look at the moon together.

For the journey with your loved one near the end of life, you both need scenery to distract you from what can be a long, hard trip. You need sights and sounds to draw out your imagination. You need rest stops to replenish your energy.

Every human life has the makings of spiritual scenery. The raw materials are home and family, culture, religion, heritage, and the experiences and traditions that make your life distinctive. No one can presume to know what will re-fresh the spirit of other weary sojourners. But spiritual scenery of one kind or another fills a universal need: it lifts our eyes to the source of strength that can help us through these most difficult times.

As on any trip, sometimes the scenery is in nature, or in events along the way that entertain or enlighten us. At other times, the most beautiful scenery is in the faces of those we love. There are countless ways to find spiritual scenery. Some of these include life review, reunions and gatherings, rituals, and religious ceremonies.

Life Review

Pausing amid the medications and clinical care to look back on life's highs and lows is like letting one of those accordion-folded chains of picture postcards fall out with all their varied views. Some of the life review postcards will be memories to treasure. Others may be snapshots we would rather forget, but they are there just the same, to be looked at once more.

Life review is simply looking back over life. It can be done formally, taking one chapter at a time from early childhood through the present. You are the scribe. You simply listen, possibly making written notes or tapes (audio or video) of the sessions when the dying one reminisces.

With someone who is weakened by illness you may find it best to look at vignettes of life, one or two at a time. You could start with childhood, on another occasion talk about schooling, later reminisce about marriage, and at another time list career events worth noting. It may be interesting to make a time line of life events and/or spiritual landmarks. There will be much to celebrate, but life review also allows room to grieve losses or perceived mistakes, to identify rifts and alienations in relationships past and present. Done early enough in the course of terminal illness, it offers chances for reconciliation and forgiveness.

During just such a life review, Gordon mentioned to the chaplain that his last wish was to find the son with whom he had lost contact twenty years earlier. The chaplain found a detective to help in the search, and it took only one day to find the son—who, as it turned out, had been searching for his father for many years. Their first visit was by telephone, but the second was face to face. Gordon fought hard to stay alive for another few days as he and his son reunited.

Life review can bring dramatic results, such as Gordon's reunion with his son, or quiet satisfaction and resolution. Life reviews can inspire families and friends to look at scrapbooks or even make new scrapbooks together at the bedside of the one who is dying. Some families make a picture collage of favorite events and people, easy to see at a glance. Life review sessions around old photos and shared memories inject the spiritual medicines of laughter and tears, joy and anguish. Treasure hunting through old keepsakes can provide hours of enjoyable memories.

JOURNALING

Reflecting in a daily journal or diary can be a handy tool of life review. While journaling in the present enables the dying one to share today's feelings, old diaries and letters and greeting cards make it easy to go back in time.

ARTISTRY

Making greeting cards from keepsakes and photos, with a personal note or favorite quote inside, is a simple way to continue communicating when other methods have become difficult. A dying child can reminisce and share through art, music, play, or puppets (talking indirectly through the puppet often is easier for children than talking directly to adults).

In a Jewish tradition, dying persons leave behind an *ethical will*—a written legacy of their central beliefs and values, their favorite poems and sayings and Scripture passages, important life lessons they have learned, recipes, advice, and good wishes for their loved ones. They may even leave instructions for those left behind, with every expectation that those instructions will be followed.

An ethical will does not need to be long or difficult to prepare. Try to write one as a spiritual exercise for yourself. Give yourself fifteen to thirty minutes. Write from your heart what you would like others to remember about you, and you will quickly see why ethical wills became such a time-honored tradition. They leave behind a record of the dying one's spiritual possessions, just as standard wills leave behind instructions for the disposition of material possessions.

The ethical will answers a comforting "yes" to the question: After I die, will anyone know I was here?

"I'VE ALWAYS WANTED TO . . ."

Sometimes, life reflection makes people who are nearing the end of life want to do something just one more time, or to do something new at least once before life passes.

If life review brings forth some special wish or longing, try to make it happen. The joy that comes from a last memory-making excursion is priceless. Most of the time such wishes are not hard to fulfill.

One woman with terminal cancer wanted to shop with her daughters just once more. They arranged a van to handle her and all her medical equipment, her daughters, and her grandchildren, and off they went for a short shopping spree.

In a hospice in England, a dying woman overheard a visiting physician say he was going to the ballet in Covent Garden that night. She exclaimed, "Oh, I always wanted to do that." He stopped what he was doing and said, "Let's do it!" Several days later he took her to the ballet, not letting her weakness, immobility, or need for supplemental oxygen get in the way. Her wish to see the Royal Ballet just once before she died was fulfilled.

The trick is to be creative and flexible. If your loved one can't manage more than an hour of activity, so be it. If Dad wants a walk along the beach but can no longer walk, take him for a ride in the car down a beach highway, push him along the harbor in a wheelchair, or—if all else fails—bring a box of sand and seashells to the room and let him run his fingers through it. The magic is in the sensation of living again, even for a moment.

Reunions and Gatherings

For those who live among caring and congenial people, family reunions and gatherings of special friends may supply some of the most vivid end-of-life scenery. Many of those who are dying find comfort in being surrounded by familiar voices talking about anything whatsoever, smelling the smells of favorite foods prepared for the crowd, being hugged and kissed by those they love, being showered with attention, and knowing that these loved ones came together just for them. Stories abound of those near death holding onto life until after some special event—perhaps a birthday party, a family reunion, a wedding, or the arrival of a new baby in the family.

Lisa, a vivacious forty-year-old nurse who had battled diabetes since childhood, was gradually dying. Her family stayed by her side in shifts—telling family stories, singing camp songs and hymns, laughing, bantering, joking. Her brother, who played the harmonica horribly, persisted in playing anyway, just as always. These reunions lifted the spirits of every family member gathered and helped them in their grief work. Family members recognized that they were connected with each other in a bond of love and laughter that would continue beyond death.

Rituals

The community of a Native American man surrounded him at his death. He heard music, drum beats, and rattling gourds. He saw vibrant colors and the familiar movements of feather fans. Incense filled the air as Prayers to the Four Directions ascended. The dying man could only move one finger and smile as these rituals took place around his deathbed. But with that one feeble gesture and faint smile, he showed his spiritual pleasure.

Rituals offer a chance, at the time of death, to heal some of the brokenness of life. In a Cherokee ritual members of the community come together to tell and retell beloved traditional stories, and together they ponder, "What is the lesson in this story?" Through the stories, they look for meaning.

You and your loved one may not have the luxury of time for life review, ethical wills, reunions, and the like. When you have only a few hours or days to walk this road, rituals can compress a lifetime of memories, experience, and meaning into a few brief but familiar acts.

Everyone has personal rituals that can provide spiritual scenery at life's end. Marta, a lifelong Roman Catholic in her early forties dying from emphysema, prayed to the Virgin Mary, particularly to Our Lady of Guadalupe, and to other saints. "My tears come out," she said about her times of meditation. Her ritual repeated an ancient and widespread tradition that came alive in her own experience.

Rituals are built in to many faith traditions, yet they can be individualized to meet the dying person's needs. You may wish to collect meaningful items (such as a copy of the Torah, Quran, or Bible, a prayer book, symbols, bells, candles, pictures or icons) on a nearby table or shelf to remind the patient of spiritual things. Catholic patients may be calmed by saying the Rosary; persons in other faith traditions can also find serenity in touching loosely strung beads as they repeat the words of prayers or other meditative passages. It is not the actual number of repetitions but the cadence, the rhythm and touch of moving the beads, that centers and comforts.

CENTERING PRAYER

A form of meditation called the "centering prayer" means, at its simplest, to pick one word (a name, an object, a feeling) that carries great spiritual meaning for you and consciously block your mind from any thought except that word. By closing your eyes and centering in silence on that one word, you allow the mind to go to a sacred place where the divine often comes to enlighten, encourage, or comfort.

Another prayer path is to read a passage from a holy text or a meditation guide and then let your mind wander back to the one phrase that "jumps out" at you with meaning at that particular moment. Repeat that phrase in your mind throughout the day, drawing strength, hope, and inspiration from it. Many believe that a higher power points you toward the words that will help you most if you open yourself to divine direction.

SIMPLE RITUALS

Rituals can be as uncomplicated as a good night kiss or hearing a child's bedtime prayers. Rituals may include a daily reflection or journal entry, a wife singing to her husband, a friend reading aloud to the one who is ill, watching a favorite TV show or classic movie together, back rubs, or eating sweet rolls and listening to favorite music while reading the Sunday paper.

A hospice musician has seen restless patients fall asleep, and even die peacefully, when she plays classical guitar or sings songs from their faith tradition. One family used water for a ritual blessing, each touching the patient's head with water and then speaking a goodbye. Rituals can be as soothing as the sound of waves lapping against the shore or as uplifting as the view of a sunset on the sea's horizon—spiritual scenery to soften a hard and often tiring approach to life's end.

Ceremonies

Alicia was only thirty-one and newly engaged to be married when she learned she had liver cancer. She and her fiancé first decided to postpone the wedding, but as time went by they changed their minds. She put her heart and soul into planning her wedding, an outdoor ceremony in a Virginia garden. There was nothing traditional about it, but it was uniquely theirs.

Two weeks later, her new husband and her family came back to the same garden for Alicia's memorial service.

Ceremonies create lasting scenes and memories both for the dying person and for all taking part in the event. Every one of the hundreds of world religions has unique religious ceremonies that mark important milestones for its followers. Whatever the rite—the laying on of hands, last rites, or Holy Communion brought to a dying Christian; prayers from the Quran for a Muslim; or reciting the traditional prayers, Psalms, and readings from the Torah for a person of the Jewish faith (to name a few)—these ceremonies convey profound meaning.

Some religious rites near the end of life require clergy assistance. Families should feel free to call their pastor, rabbi, imam, chaplain, or other worship leader, but only if they know that the dying person wants (or would want) it. The spiritual companion and the person near the end of life, along with family and friends, can plan these rites and sometimes even conduct the ceremonies.

Sometimes it is comforting for the dying person to plan the funeral. A twelve-year-old boy named Kyle asked his mom to help him plan his service. He predicted he would be there with them in spirit, watching his grand finale. Kyle wanted to be buried in his Texas A&M jacket and chose a casket in the A&M school colors (silver with maroon lining). He picked out a burial plot at the edge of the cemetery, under a tree next to a field of grazing cows, and selected a poem for a friend to read. Kyle's friends from the local police department led the funeral procession and provided a police dog at the cemetery, as he requested. Finally, Kyle specified that he did not want to be transported by a hearse but in the family car, wrapped in a comforter from his own bed. He stayed busy planning and then savored those plans until he died.

Whatever brings peace, whatever brings closure, whatever gives cause for love and celebration, should be arranged if it is possible. Those occasions are the life scenery we will always cherish.

Don't forget to take pictures! Cameras may seem oddly out of place as a person nears death, and the person may not want pictures taken, but if the person is willing, the pictures will be priceless later on. Even at the time, taking pictures may honor the person who is dying as one still very present, alive, and loved.

Spiritual scenery provides an oasis, a resting place, a party, or an emotional high as you travel with your companion toward the end of life. Rituals, reunions, life review, and religious ceremonies have the power to lift us up and to give us strength for the road ahead. Let these tools take you and your loved one to higher ground, and anticipate views from lookout points along the way.

4 *For Weary Travelers*

As a spiritual companion, you will sometimes feel tired beyond belief. You may wonder why you are so exhausted when you have only been sitting by the side of the dying one, watching the hours and days tick by. Death can be relentlessly exhausting, both for the one who is leaving and for the spiritual companion. The travelers are weary, longing for closure on the one hand, yet dreading what will bring it on the other.

Blessedly, there are comforts of body and soul for you weary ones. The restful ideas presented here harvest the best fruits of people who have worked with the dying and their loved ones for many years. They are divided into comforts for those near the end of life and comforts for their companions, but they are interchangeable. Tired is tired.

Comforts for the Dying

Preferences for physical comforts are highly individual, yet we hope that something in these pages will help you and your traveling companion claim a measure of peace and solace as life comes to a close. Let the one who is dying lead you.

A grieving husband climbed up onto his dying wife's hospital bed and leaned down to kiss her. Their eldest daughter, who was sitting on the other side of the bed, said to her mother, "Do you want to give Dad a hug?" Her mom's eyes opened wide, so the daughter picked up her paralyzed arm and placed it over his shoulder. The husband whispered to his wife, "This is how we started out," and his wife, who had not spoken for over a day, replied, "The first family!"

Touch is a spiritual gift and a powerful antidote to suffering. African Americans put a high priority on touching the one who is terminally ill, as do many other cultures. You may simply hold the hand of the one who is dying. One man recalled that he slept beside his mom with his arm around her for several weeks before she died.

For touch to comfort, a person needs fresh bedding and a clean body not plagued by pain or nausea. One hospice nurse reminded us that it is hard for a patient to be spiritually at peace when his or her physical needs are not met first. Favorite soft pajamas warm and fragrant out of the dryer, a puffy quilt or coverlet, soft slippers, even a horseshoe-shaped pillow to anchor the weak person's head are simple ways to provide comfort through touch. (One man would not be separated from his pajamas and slippers with golf balls on them. One middle-aged woman, to her family's amusement, insisted on wearing her Yankees baseball cap to the very end and even to her grave.)

The Furry Touch

A touch does not necessarily have to be a human touch. A writer's dog lay by her side in the hospice where she could stroke and be nuzzled by the animal as she died. A beloved cat knows just where to curl up at the bend of the knee or along the back to become a living hot water bottle. Companion animals give and receive love through touch, and they need comforting, too. But even a visiting animal, trained by one of the many pet therapy programs now supporting hospitals and hospices, can give a warm touch and elicit a smile.

Even inanimate pets can comfort.

Kevin, a terminally ill teenager, had seemed aloof. Many hospital staff members (and even his relatives) chalked it up to typical adolescent behavior. Congregations around Kevin's city had donated small, stuffed lambs for distribution to young patients. Members of the churches and synagogues held blessing ceremonies at which they promised to pray for the children who would receive the stuffed pets. Kevin was given a lamb figurine rather than the usual plush version because the chaplain, trying to be sensitive to his age, thought a toddler's toy would insult him. When Kevin realized the difference, he protested, "I want a soft lamb, not this!" The stuffed lamb seemed to help Kevin to soften and begin welcoming conversation.

Tips for Touching

One dying woman lamented, "How can anyone love me when I can't do anything? I don't look good. I don't smell good. Why should they want to be around me?" There are many little ways in which you can offer the gift of touch to your dying companion who feels untouchable.

Bathe the person often and gently.

Between baths, you can freshen the person's dry skin

with a damp washcloth or one of the misting facial products available at any drug store.

For the person who would welcome it (not all would!), try massaging hands and feet, ever so gently, possibly using lotions but remembering that perfumes may bother sensitive noses.

A person who has never liked being touched may find comfort in the pressure of your hand on the side of the bed, being turned in the bed, or a playful but gentle nudge on the shoulder.

Hair brushing, pillow plumping, or rubbing shoulders, back, or temples lightly usually feels wonderful to one who is ill.

Even a finger or two on the patient's gown may serve as a physical but nonintrusive reminder of your presence.

One hospice physician believes there is a very real phenomenon called "skin hunger." Human nature longs for touch. Skin hunger in infants who have not been cuddled or handled enough influences their emotional health for a lifetime. Skin hunger also occurs in the ill and elderly whose friends and family withdraw from touching because of their distaste for the person's physical condition or fear of contracting a disease.

Only touch can satisfy skin hunger. The spiritual companion who provides a dying loved one with ample touching offers a valuable spiritual blessing.

A man dying of AIDS lay still and depressed in his dark room, with all window shades pulled down. Then, one of his spiritual companions touched him on the shoulder, lightly, as if to say, "I am here with you." He looked up, welcoming, from his solitary confinement. "Nobody touches me," *he said. The touch alone had a miraculous effect. In days to come, he had the window shades up, the light on, and music playing. One touch reconnected him to life.*

SIGHT

What can lift the spirits more than the sight of someone you love coming through the door, the flicker of a fire in the fireplace, or colorful flowers blossoming in your garden outside the window?

The old saying "You are a sight for sore eyes" rings true on the spiritual journey near the end of life. People are generally the most welcome sights for eyes weary with illness. Just seeing an old friend's face, even with no words spoken, can bring spiritual comfort in the midst of pain.

All kinds of art and photographs; videos; gifts of nature such as agates, flowers, or seashells; or aquariums can provide soothing visual relief from the hard road. Keep in mind your loved one's personal aesthetic tastes when you choose visual gifts.

If there is a pleasant view from the window—or even a passing scene, people coming and going or children playing—try to position the bed so the patient can visually participate in the world outside.

A woman tells of sitting by her dying father's side, trying in vain to lift him from his deep depression. Nothing seemed to stir him; no memory brought a smile or a softening of his gloom. Suddenly the tree outside his window became vibrant as a flock of migrating goldfinches settled onto its branches. Father and daughter watched without moving or talking. As the golden cloud lifted and flew away she looked back at her dad and saw him beaming.

In the Looking Glass

Another important sight for sore eyes is what the patient sees in the mirror. One man who had only days to live wanted a fresh haircut; his barber came to his home and gave him a royal shave and haircut just to his liking. Looking better made him feel better. A stylish woman wanted her nails done. Why not? Her nails had always been one of the indulgences she allowed herself. Most patients find a shampoo, even a dry bed shampoo, to be incredibly cheering.

It may not be possible to love how you look at the end of life, but there are definitely ways to make the reflected image more satisfying. Help the patient feel as attractive as possible under the circumstances. Assure your loved one that he or she is beautiful in your eyes.

Guided Imagery

One of the most powerful comforts of sight at any point in life can happen, oddly enough, with the eyes closed. It is called guided imagery. Comfortably positioned (either sitting or lying down), eyes shut, the patient is verbally led by another down an imagined pathway that leads to the beach, to a favorite getaway, or to some other mental sanctuary. There the weary one rests for a time, walking the imaginary beach or sitting on a garden bench, by a fire, on a mountain peak, or wherever the image has led. Then, moving from the toes up all the way to the top of the head, the guide coaches the patient to relax the entire body, breathing deep, long breaths, to linger in this state of relaxation awhile, and gradually to move back to the present.

With practice, guided imagery can be a self-guided tour, but generally the person using it needs to have a few sessions with a leader, or listen to a tape, before going it alone.

SOUND

Sound is, reportedly, the last of the senses to leave the human body. People who have returned from near-death comas say they remember hearing sounds and voices. Persons who are otherwise unresponsive may give a squeeze or a faint smile when hearing the voice of someone they love, a favorite tune, or a sentence that is meaningful to them.

Speech

Assume that your loved one is present with you and can hear you clearly, right to the last instant of life. The greatest spiritual gift associated with sound is speaking directly to (not about) the person. Never talk as if the person, however near the end of life, is already gone. The sweetest sound of all is the sound of inclusion—in conversation, jokes and thoughts, decision-making, prayer, and shared feelings of every kind.

A multilingual person who is dying surely will treasure the sound of the first, childhood tongue—if you don't know the language, perhaps you can find someone who does. The soothing cadences of passages from a holy book, a novel, poetry, or even the daily newspaper, when read out loud, are likely to be calming.

Those are the sounds of life.

Music

The rhythms and tunes of music almost always communicate movingly in the last days of life. Your loved one may retreat to a place that is beyond language or be too exhausted to sort out the meanings of words and sentences. Talking may be painful or simply impossible. But music has the power to reach into those final places, to soothe and bring peace, but also to enliven the mood. Cheerful music with a beat is not necessarily inappropriate.

A retired pastor who was dying had always loved singing hymns, old and new. His children began to sing hymns to him as he slipped in and out of consciousness, and his response was so positive that they sang themselves hoarse through his last three days. He could even indicate preferences; he turned his eyes upwards, beamed, and feebly lifted his good arm during hymns of praise, but merely smiled politely during the sad, weepy ones.

What kind of music do you like? It doesn't matter. Whether you play CDs, sing, or invite a musician or grandchild to perform, choose the kind of music that the *patient* has always loved. It could be opera or bluegrass, cool jazz or rock 'n' roll. Hymns, symphonies, folk music, oratorios, school songs, country laments, or polkas—even a harmonica played badly (see the story of Lisa in Chapter 3)—can bring joy. If you are at home, play or sing as loudly as the person seems to want, but respect other patients' need for quiet and keep the volume down if you are in a hospice, hospital, or nursing home.

Music is very important to many people. If you don't already know the patient's tastes and preferences, find out. It will make the difference between adding to the distress (by playing music the person hates) and lifting spirits. For example, if you are giving companionship to a dying uncle who has expensive audio equipment, music from a boom box will put his teeth on edge. If possible, set up his best equipment in the room — just make sure you place the speakers a good distance from the wall!

TASTE AND SMELL

Living fully until death means using all of the senses. Often the loved ones of a person who is nearing death recognize the importance of sight, hearing, and touch, but forget the value of taste and smell.

Flavors

Just a little taste of something familiar can go a long, long way. A dropper full of coffee at the very end of life meant a lot to one dying man; a teaspoonful of cranberry juice caused a woman who was otherwise unresponsive to say "Mmmm" contentedly. A young woman approaching death asked her friend for home-fried chicken, apologizing, "I know that's a lot of trouble." Her companion answered honestly, "Yes it is, but you're worth it, and I think you would do the same for me."

If ever there is time for a little indulgence, this is it. A 78-year-old man had suffered a massive stroke and was steadily (but very slowly) losing his life force. His grown children, knowing he had always loved chocolate, brought a box to his room in the nursing home — but his wife took it away because "it's bad for his heart." The children saw the disappointment in his eyes and were dumbfounded. Obviously eating a whole box of chocolate would have caused him greater discomfort, but he had never been a greedy man.

How few of his little joys remain, they wondered. What harm could a little taste of chocolate do him now?

Aromas

The aroma of familiar food coming from the kitchen may comfort the one who is ill as well as the companions. One family prepared Kosher chicken soup so their Jewish mother could smell it bubbling on the stove. It may not be important that the patient eat the food; just the smell of it is satisfying, as is watching other loved ones enjoy a good meal. Sometimes people who are terminally ill worry whether their loved ones will take care of themselves and are reassured to see them eat.

Sometimes fragrance can bring comfort. Lavender and eucalyptus often soothe nausea in cancer patients. There are lavender and other scented sprays for bed linens.

Mild herbal or regular teas provide scent, taste, touch, and ritual; just be sure to note the effects of caffeine on your loved one and avoid it if it causes anxiety or sleeplessness.

The patient may have favorite scented soaps, shampoos, lotions, colognes, or perfumes.

Breath mints and breath sprays can be helpful and refreshing to counteract a dry or sour mouth.

It is important, though, to be sensitive about individual responses to scents. If you smoke, be sure you have shampooed your hair and put on clean clothes, because the smell of stale smoke may be objectionable or even nauseating to a person who is medicated, taking radiation treatments, or just plain sick. If your loved one is allergic to or intolerant of perfumes—or just doesn't like them—their presence can cause migraine headaches, nausea, breathing problems, or simple annoyance. In that case you will want to rely on natural aromas such as brewing coffee, sun-dried sheets, or freshly baked bread for pleasure.

COMFORT FROM A DISTANCE

Even when you are separated by many miles and cannot directly offer some of these sensory pleasures to the one who is dying, there are many ways to comfort from afar. You will come up with your own ideas for things you can do to ease a person's mind and buoy the spirits, such as the following:

Regular telephone calls
Letters and encouraging cards
Assurance of your thoughts (even specifying a daily time devoted to thinking of the patient)
Care packages of things to please the senses (tapes and CDs, a soft fleece pullover, favorite candy if it's allowable, pressed flowers from your garden)

E-mail can provide even more frequent long-distance companionship. Through the Internet you can send daily visual reminders by attaching digital photos of yourself, your family, and other people, places, and pets of interest to the loved one.

Whatever comforts you send from a distance, keep them coming steadily. It's all too easy, when you first hear the bad news, to send an avalanche of gifts and messages that gradually dribble down to little or nothing. Better to send little messages that don't take much time—a scribbled "I'm thinking of you," a clipping from a newspaper, a postcard with a few words on the back, a three-minute telephone call, an e-mailed photograph—than to start something you can't keep up. If necessary, preaddress and stamp a boxful of envelopes and set them by your front door. Decide what will be realistic; write it on your calendar and do it consistently.

Companion Comforts

An elderly, dying woman named Amelia was sobbing when the chaplain walked into her room. "My granddaughter doesn't love me anymore. She left mad, and she's not coming back."

It turned out the granddaughter had reached her limit under the strains of providing care to her grandmother. She felt she had to get out for a while, and in due time she came back. She never intended not to return. Before the afternoon was out, the whole family was happy to surround the grandmother for a family photo that even included the dog. Amelia was delighted someone still wanted to take her picture and that her granddaughter wasn't mad at her. She felt loved once more.

ACCEPTING LIMITS

Lessons in this little vignette are important for all spiritual companions. At some point, unless the dying happens very quickly, you will wear out. Your well of energy, and even of caring, is not inexhaustible. You need to refresh your supply of physical and psychic vitality before the well runs dry. Amelia's granddaughter did the right thing to get away, but she probably should have left before sending out signals that could be read as anger.

MINI-BREAKS

All companions need an oasis of solitude now and then. If the care of the one who is dying does not allow for long breaks, take mini-breaks.

A trip to the grocery store, a walk with your dog, a bubble bath, reading the newspaper or E-mail all can be therapeutic.

Step outside at night and look at the stars.

Take a nap snuggled under a favorite quilt with a soft pillow at your head. Put a recliner or cot by the bedside of your loved one expressly for that purpose.

Read a good book while you sit with your loved one.

Play solitaire or a game on a laptop computer.

FOOD AND EXERCISE

Put a pot of soup on the stove and enjoy the smell and taste of comfort food, or pop down to the hospital cafeteria for a nutritious hot snack. Eat healthy food. Rely on the endorphins of exercise (endorphins are proven mental spirit lifters induced by physical activity).

SHARING THE BURDEN

Discuss your situation with a trusted friend all along the way. Talk to the spiritual presence that sustains you. Feel free to lament, to protest, or to be angry in those conversations. Be honest about how you are feeling. Attend a worship service and feel buoyed by your faith community. Ask people to pray for you, and lean on their support.

Lean on your family members. This experience can repair torn relationships and strengthen the family to go on without the loved one, or it can cause further estrangement. Try for the happier of the two outcomes.

ACCEPTING HELP

Do not refuse any reasonable offer of help. If you have a hard time asking for help, put a well-organized friend to the task of giving out assignments. When people offer to help, they generally mean it. They may feel helpless to know what you need and will truly appreciate a chance to do something concrete. You could tell them favorite foods you would enjoy or household chores that need doing. Mowing the lawn, catching up a few loads of laundry, or cleaning the kitchen are easy enough tasks that even mere acquaintances will take joy in doing during your time of need.

UTILIZING VOLUNTEERS

If you are fortunate enough to be supported by a hospice team, ask if there is a volunteer available to help you. One woman asked a volunteer to be with her terminally ill father while she and her husband went to a concert. They reported that the outing, and the intimacy of a date, gave them extra energy to see her father through his last several days. A daughter asked the women's circle at her mother's church to "stop praying for Mom, get over here and do something to help!"

A volunteer is as much a gift to the one who is ill as to you, infusing new energy, new interest, new stories, new activities, and even new fun. You may be too tired to play cards or read a story, listen to a CD or watch a favorite old movie, but the volunteer is fresh and available to do anything that makes the ill person feel better. It is amazing to watch a dying patient rally just from the knowledge that a volunteer will be coming. People who are ill need these new faces and unwearied companions as badly as their companions need the break. You may tire of each other on this journey before it is over; both of you will benefit from short breaks. Volunteers are happy to supply this welcome respite.

PROFESSIONAL HELP

If a volunteer is not available, a hired caregiver can take over for a while. At the end of her father's life Zoë, a busy career woman with a family of her own, tried desperately to attend his every hour. The hospice nurse finally told her, "I will tell you when you need to stay the night, when death is that close. I know these things. Until then, why don't you have a sitter come so you can sleep at home?" Zoë followed the advice, and when the nurse told her it was time to stay, she had the energy to be fully present at her father's death. Admittedly, it was possible that Zoë would not arrive in time and he would already be gone—but it was doing her father no good to have a wilted, forlorn, and exhausted companion at his side.

GIVING AND RECEIVING CARE

Spiritual companionship is a two-way street of giving and receiving care.

Caroline, attending to her mother, Dottie, before death, experienced increasing anxiety and emotional distress. At last, she realized that she was longing for her mother to take care of her. She told Dottie how she would miss her mothering, and Dottie, though very weak, stroked Caroline's hair as she had done many times through the years. In that moment they wept and cared for each other's sadness.

GUILT AND RESENTMENT

Sometimes companions struggle with the demands of the journey. This is normal. You may feel resentful or even jealous of all the attention showered on the one who is dying. "This dying. This isn't easy for me either," you think. It may seem the dying process is going to take forever, and you feel guilty for feeling that way. No matter how hard or fast you work, the needs of the dying person outdistance your best efforts, and the job seems endless.

REALISTIC EXPECTATIONS

Whenever you can, give yourself grace. Remember again that you are a companion, not a leader, and you are not responsible for the timing or the final outcome.

EASING UP

Tell people your limits. Realize that we all need refueling, particularly for such a journey. There may be a point of emotional and spiritual fatigue that incapacitates you. When you feel yourself nearing that point, stop short of it and rest. Become self-aware—both for your own sake and for the sake of your fellow traveler.

HONESTY

The only way a spiritual journey at the end of life can progress positively is for both traveling companions to be honest. When you need a break from one another, say so. You will need to attend to your other life when possible. Bills continue to pile up, your job may call you away from your loved one, children need attention, and other family and friends want some of your time occasionally.

Trouble along the Road

It is tempting to idealize the one who is dying. But people die as they live, with their original personalities. Persons who have been angry in life will use anger to cope with death. If your loved one has always had a sharp tongue, expect some barks. At other times, medication or illness may change the person in uncomfortable ways. A formerly stalwart stroke victim may cry all the time, or an active and involved executive may become passive and disinterested under the influence of powerful drugs. Dying does not necessarily bring out the best in a person. This is not within your power to change.

An elderly, highly critical, controlling mother had been particularly tough on her son Charles all day long. Even from her hospital bed this woman, weak as she was, could do damage. In early evening the chaplain saw Charles standing dejectedly outside the room. "I know my mother is dying, and I've tried to get close to her," he sighed, "but it is so difficult." The chaplain went into the room with Charles. The old woman was clearly near death. She motioned Charles to come closer, said something in his ear, and then died. "What did she tell you?" the chaplain asked expectantly. "She told me to tuck in my shirt and zip up my fly."

What if the dying person is the combative partner of a deeply troubled relationship? An antisocial brother who has been in and out of prison? A mean old rattlesnake of a grandfather? A mother who is cold and uncaring, who has criticized and humiliated her children for a lifetime? A drug or alcohol addict who can no longer process information or follow the sequence of a conversation?

The mean old rattlesnake of a grandfather may still strike. The callous mom may find fault to the very end. If so, you will never find out if your efforts touched a soft spot or sparked a fond memory. You can only hope, and take consolation in the peace of mind that comes from doing what you could do. Spiritual companionship calls for acceptance, but not for taking abuse. You may need to set boundaries, such as making clear that abusive language is not an option. You might say, "I'm having a hard time being with you right now. I'm leaving, but I'll be back." Sometimes taking a break defuses anger and gives a chance for a fresh start.

What if your loved one is an Alzheimer's patient who has lost all memory and recognition? For your own peace of mind you may want to be present, provide some creature comforts, perhaps play some music that you know the person used to enjoy. Peace of mind may be all you will get in such situations. You may never know if your presence held off a demon of loneliness or fear, if your occasional "remember when" transported the suffering one to a happier time. You may not be able to discern if a person with dementia will even recognize that you were there.

The spiritual journey near the end of life is likely to be wearying, even when it is very brief. Bone-numbing fatigue results from the high emotional toll of your situation. Forgive yourself for not being able to provide everything you would like to give. This trip can sap the strength and spirit of even the most dedicated and loving spiritual companion.

The same comforts that help the weary one traveling toward death can help you as you travel alongside. They can bring the awareness that both of you are surrounded by what is called in the Hebrew language *shekhinah*, the cloud of divine presence that will hover about you until weariness is no more.

5 Parting Ways

It was almost over. The grandfather's life seemed like a candle about to flicker out. His grandson, Jonathan, who was twenty-two and had always been unable to walk due to cerebral palsy, was saying good night to Pop, his lifelong buddy, for the last time. "I'll be able to run to you when I see you in heaven," Jonathan said. "And I'll welcome you with open arms," Pop replied softly.

The time arrives for parting ways. The spiritual journey near the end of life may seem endless at some points, but it will end. "Parting is such sweet sorrow," wrote Shakespeare. But even during the last hours of the journey, there is spiritual work that still can be done.

Peace is the goal—peace for the one who is dying and peace for the ones who are left to live a bit longer. Just as we packed to begin the spiritual journey near the end of life, now we have unpacking to do. This passage requires no baggage, no cumbersome loads, and no heavy burdens.

Unpacking Life's Baggage

A caller to a radio talk show recently said, somewhat flippantly, "You'll never see a moving van following a hearse." A person's possessions, interests, hobbies, and life's work may be infused with precious memories and profound meaning, but at death they all must be left behind.

Sometimes the one who is dying wants to give some possessions to particular friends and family members. You can help with this task.

Your loved one may want to see someone for the last time—ask if there is anyone you can track down and bring in for a final visit. A former spouse may be on the list. By all means extend the invitation, for the ex-spouse shares the life story of the person who is dying, often a story that includes children.

Peace seeking for the dying frequently involves tying up loose ends from many chapters of life. Help that to happen if you can.

Set your companion free from "getting that last thing done." One elderly man had always made a point of not doing his taxes until the last possible minute. His death approached at the end of March. It was sweet freedom for him to hear that a trusted friend was taking care of his tax return. Releasing the dying from the details of life can greatly assist them in letting go and finding spiritual peace.

Giving Permission to Go

Tell your loved one that you will be okay. One way to say it might be, "You don't have to stay for us. I love you enough to let you go, and we will be all right." A woman told her father, "Daddy, I feel like you are at the gates of heaven this very minute. If you want to, walk on through. I'll take care of Mom. We can make it; you have taught us how."

Reconciliation

At the end of life, most people long to experience reconciliation with others and with their higher power. If that means offering a chance to repent, please listen earnestly and don't rush to pardon too quickly. There is healing in earnest repentance. If it means saying, "I forgive you for things you have done, and I hope you forgive me," then say it. If it means calling in a pastor or spiritual leader to hear a last confession, make it happen. Family members are often not the best ones to hear confessions. The dying person may not want to share past shortcomings with you, and you may not want to hear them. Allow the faith community to listen and absolve when it is more appropriate.

Last rituals aid in this reconciliation. In the Jewish tradition, for example, the Vidui (the final confessional prayer) is said either by the dying person or by companions. In the Buddhist faith, the dying are led by a spiritual guide who reads aloud from *The Tibetan Book of Living and Dying*. The spiritual guide tells the family when it is time to let go. Every Muslim, or someone else in the person's stead, must utter a statement of faith at the last breath. There are countless liturgical rites for dying, many including readings from holy books and prayers.

The rituals around death are as myriad as the cultures and faith traditions of the world. But the point of them is the same: to help people die in spiritual peace—forgiven, loved, and free to leave this life.

Religious rituals can influence whether the dying person accepts pain medication. Some want to be alert at all costs in order to profess their faith at the end. Some want to drift toward death peacefully. Buddhists, for instance, believe that a peaceful state at death has bearing on what you will be in your next life. If at all possible, the wishes of the dying need to be honored, no matter how unsettling they may be to the family and clinical team. This is no time for the dying to sacrifice so the living can be comfortable.

When a little boy of the Muslim faith neared death, his mother raged at Allah for taking her son from her. The boy had wanted to say his daily prayers with her, but she refused. The chaplain talked with the boy, in such a way that she could overhear them, about his wish that she would pray with him again because he wanted to be with her in Paradise. When she heard that, she came into the room but would not lift her hands as is customary. The next day she lifted her hands a little. On the third day she lifted her hands fully and joined them in prayer.

You may be in a spiritual, religious, emotional, or political place far from your companion's position. The dying person may be angry, despondent, or frustrated while you are filled with hope. Your loved one may want to hear a song of praise or a poem of thanks for all life's blessings when you are feeling cynical and low. Try to oblige such requests, regardless of your current spiritual vantage point. It is a good thing to do. You will have time, later, to sort out your own feelings. Now is the only time there is for the one who is dying.

Holy Silence

There will probably be a space of time—hours or days or weeks—when your dying loved one is (or appears to be) unresponsive. Spiritual companionship continues in that holy silence. Some believe that the person who is dying has turned inward, expending the last little flicker of energy on soul work. How good to hold the hand of the one who is doing that hard work. In the Buddhist tradition, the spiritual companion experiences unity with the dying one by breathing in the same rhythm when words are spoken no more.

This period of silence may be a time for you to reflect on your own spiritual journey, how you have changed and grown from this experience. It may be time just to sit still and rest.

Joshua remembers vividly what it was like to wait in silence during the last hours of his father's life. He calls it a vigil. His father hung on for three hours, then seemed about to leave, then lived another two hours. Feeling a bit helpless, Joshua sat back down, leaning forward, resting his elbows on his knees. He noticed that it was still quite warm outside and the crickets and assorted late summer insects were beginning their evening humming and chanting. The whole moment, he remembers, felt very familiar. He wrote down the experience: "I went back in my mind to when I was a kid, when my father and I spent August afternoons at the edge of the local river, bottom fishing with night crawlers, waiting for Bluegill, Sunfish, or an occasional Largemouth or Catfish. I would find a Y-shaped branch and poke it into the ground to hold up my fishing pole. After casting my worm ball, letting it sink to the river bottom, and resting the pole on the branch, I'd watch—in a boyish trance—my pole and its line stretching out into the water. . . . Any apparent movement caught my attention, and I would pull myself off the ground and rush over to my pole, ready to set the hook in what might be a lunker on the other end. But before grabbing the pole, uncertain of what was really happening, I'd look back to my father. Invariably he'd say to me, 'Sit down, be patient, you'll know it when you've really got one.' And though it took decades, I was glad that we were there again, in late August, quietly and patiently waiting together."

Suspending Disbelief

People who are dying may see angels and other visions. Many of these are comforting; some can be frightening. Who are we to dispute their word?

A little boy who had an organ transplant saw angels coming for him and told his mother that he wanted to go with them. The next day, he died unexpectedly. His mother believed that his angels were real, and she took great comfort from his vision.

An elderly man saw two young men no one else could see at the door. A grandmother who longed to see her newborn granddaughter before she died heard the child crying in the next room, when in fact mother and baby were still en route. A four-year-old boy with AIDS saw angels flying around the corners of the room. "They are making a very special place for me," he said. "I'm going to be okay."

Sometimes people see other loved ones who have died before and converse with them. "Don't you see her?" they may ask. You can give an honest but accepting reply, such as, "No, I can't see her, but I believe you do."

If the dying person perceives, as a woman named Graciela did, that she will have wings like a bird in heaven and be able to fly to people who are crying or in need, this is not a time to challenge her belief. You may not agree with her, but you can defer to her. Heaven is heaven as she defines it. This is her time, and she is the only one whose opinion matters. Your time will come. Just listen and affirm their perceived visions if they are pleasant; soothe their fears if they are not.

Don't rule out the possibility that during this period of waiting and sadness, you may have your own visions and sense of being attended by angels or a divine presence. You may rush to find explanations, but why? Why not relax and open your mind to welcome these visitations? They will strengthen and encourage you and remind you that you are not alone on this path.

Sometimes the angels come in human form, bringing food or companionship or supplying energy you just don't have. Receive them thankfully. In one rabbi's telling of the biblical story of Ruth, Ruth comforts her mother-in-law, Naomi, who is bereaved of a husband and two sons. Ruth says to Naomi, "Don't try to take hold of God's hand; take hold of mine. I will help you until you can reach God again."

Letting Go

One Sunday a retired teacher suffered a stroke in church. Doctors determined that brain death had already occurred by the time her daughter arrived at the hospital. To the pastor who broke the sad news she protested, "But God can heal!" The preacher said, "God may have already spoken." The daughter retorted, "Well, God didn't speak to ME!" With a smile the pastor told her, "Next time I talk to God, I'll tell God never to do anything without asking you first." The daughter realized at once that she was not in charge of her mother's death and approved the removal of life support as soon as she had said farewell to her mother.

You may think you have prepared yourself for letting go, but you may be surprised at how difficult it is. Usually someone—a chaplain, a friend, your pastor or spiritual leader, or another family member—will help you to release your companion when the time comes.

A gift of spiritual peace often comes at this time from a source beyond yourself.

Saying Goodbye

You have been a faithful spiritual companion, and the journey has been rich and memorable. As with every meaningful life experience, goodbye is the hardest part. It is necessary to feel closure, and it is necessary to go on to another day. Whether the person who is dying is still interacting with you or lies in a silent inner world, continue to say the things you need to say once more: "I love you." "I will miss you." "I will never forget you." "I am so proud of you." "I have been so blessed to have you in my life." "You have cared for me so much, and I appreciate it." Use your own words and your own feelings. Say goodbye in such a way that you will never have to think, "I wish I had told him . . ." or "I wish I had let her know. . . ."

LOVE AND TEARS

Love lasts. It doesn't end with your loved one's death. Share love freely as you say your goodbyes. Share tears freely, too. The anguish you feel at parting is not yours alone. The dying person you love shares your pain.

Trying to hold back tears only traps the pain of loss inside. Tears are a gift of release and healing—use them freely throughout the journey near the end of life. To see you cry gives your companion permission to cry as well. Voice your struggles out loud. Proclaim your pain at having to live with this loss.

A CHILD'S GOODBYE

Children need to say goodbye in their own way. Prepare them for what the dying person looks like. Then let them come in if they wish. A little kiss, a pat, a hug, a spoken "goodbye" or "I love you" brings comfort to their hearts, which are hurting, too.

DYING ALONE

Your spiritual companion may very well die when you aren't present. You're likely to feel upset because you wanted so much to be there. Try to remember all the time you invested in the entire journey. A chaplain reassured one grieving widow, who attended her husband continually for weeks but returned from a short break to find he had died: "It is the past fifty years that mattered, not the last fifteen minutes."

A hospice nurse told one daughter keeping midnight vigil with her mother that often the dying feel such a strong bond to their spouses and children that they are unable to let go in their presence. The ones they are leaving hold them too tightly to this life. She said that it is very common for people to die when family members finally go home for a rest. She had seen it happen again and again.

Safe Passage

At the end, all we can do as spiritual companions is to commit our loved one to journey onward safely to a destination beyond our human understanding. We watch this real, living person slowly disappear from our view. In the end it is a solitary crossing. We must turn back to life again, though it is a changed life. A loved one cannot be replaced by anyone else. You go on, but you carry with you the memory of your trip and of your beloved fellow traveler.

A Sacred Journey

The journey near the end of life is sacred. To choose to be a spiritual companion to someone on that road is an act of love and compassion. Moving in time with one who is dying means setting aside your own pace and agenda.

The rewards for your sacrifice are considerable. Death is a great teacher, the dying its disciples. They help us realize what is important, and they point us toward life's true meanings. They light the way for our lives and better prepare us for our own deaths.

UNPREDICTABLE TIMING

The spiritual companion and the one who is dying realize at some point that the timing of the trip is not really in their control. They travel toward a destination that they cannot see clearly, on a schedule not of their choosing.

A dying man asked his son, "How much longer? How much longer?" The son could only reply, "I don't know, I'm sorry." Another family member overheard the father, who was no longer communicating verbally to anyone else, say to himself, "Why am I still here? I don't have time for this."

In contrast, the father of a young woman who was dying asked her if they could plant a tree in memory of her life so that her children could see it blossom and grow and remember planting it with her. She responded, "Don't memorialize me quite yet; I'm still alive."

This journey may not end as you expected. Your loved one may die sooner than anyone thought. A second, seemingly unrelated illness or event such as pneumonia, heart attack, or stroke can snatch life away before the original disease has advanced to the point of death. People with a terminal diagnosis sometimes commit suicide. Or, after life support has been removed, the dying one may linger far longer than you imagined possible. You have no control over the timing of your loved one's departure.

As a physician, Bob had attended many deaths. Now his own father was dying, and in his final two days was still directing his own life. "No feeding tubes, no ICU, no antibiotics," he commanded.

Bob's mother, who suffered from early Alzheimer's disease, at times was tearful and at other times would sit with a goofy sort of grin—sad, then perplexed. Bob took her out of the room, and she became tearful again. "That's quite a drama we're watching," she said. "Yes, it is," he replied. She asked, "And who are the actors in this play?" Bob answered, "Dad's your husband and my father, and he's one of the actors. And I'm Bob, your son, and I'm one of the actors, and the doctor is one, and you're my mother—I guess you are in the play too." And she said, "Okay. Does the play always have the same ending?" Bob wasn't sure how to answer that one. "Well, yes, I guess we all have to die sometime." His mother seemed to take the news calmly. "Oh," she said, "Who wrote the play?" Bob thought for a minute, "I guess God did."

As a spiritual companion, you do not take away the mystery of the journey, but you can help lighten the darkness.

"We are the arms of God," a Jewish saying goes.

You can provide comfort when weariness sets in. You can help the dying person to see the spiritual scenery along the way. You somehow gather the courage to part ways. You hope for your loved one's safe passage to the unknown.

Having learned some of what is useful for spiritual companionship near the end of life, you may be able to free your creativity and learn far more on your own than in these pages. You have already satisfied the main requirement for a spiritual caregiver: You are present, and you keep showing up.

From your presence, the one you love who is dying gains blessed gifts—the gift of being heard, the gift of presence, the gift of empowerment to keep on living to the end. By necessity, death is something a person must do alone, but you have offered your hand to hold and your spiritual companionship along the way.

In the opening paragraphs of the handbook you met Doug, suffering from a malignant spinal tumor, drawing his feelings as he lay dying. Doug's first sketches during his time at the hospice were full of color, vivid with details of nature's scenery. Near the end, in every picture Doug drew two birds flying together. Sometimes the pair was off in the distance, and in other artworks the birds loomed large in the foreground.

Doug's last drawing was sketchy and faint. The image was abstract—could be a wave, could be the beginning of a mountain, could be a cloud, but quite certainly there were no birds. Perhaps he sensed that it was time to take flight alone. As Doug soared away in death, his spiritual companions watched him go. Because of the spiritual ties strengthened by their journey together, death could not take him very far from them at all.

We wish such a journey for you and your loved one. We hope that there will be spiritual awakenings and comforts along the way. May peace follow you wherever you go.

6 *Coming Home*

The journey back home alone after losing a loved one is one of the loneliest of life's experiences. The heart is often broken, the body numb with fatigue, the tears seemingly endless. Reminders seem to be everywhere of the one who has died and the void left.

It is time for the spiritual companion to rest, to take comfort in remembering, to share feelings with friends, clergy, and counselors or in helpful bereavement support groups.

Give yourself the gift of patience, please. The realization that everything you experience—the fatigue, the varied physical symptoms, even feeling the presence of the one who has died or hearing his or her voice again—all these things are part of "coming home."

Returning to "normal" life after journeying as a spiritual companion to one who is dying is a long and slow process. People who try to hurry through the grieving process usually do so unsuccessfully. Those who try to detour around grief often hit huge roadblocks later in life that send them back to face the feelings they tried to avoid.

Now spiritual companionship can take on new meaning for you. Perhaps it is finding someone who is also grieving, who can truly empathize with how you feel. Perhaps, now that you have time again, it is time to seek to expand your inventory of spiritual tools that you can use throughout life (journal if you haven't before, for example, or add a time for inspirational reading in your day; seek a closer relationship with your divine power). The next time a spiritual crisis comes up for you or someone you love, you will be more prepared.

Then wait. A day almost inevitably comes when the pain of loss diminishes and life seems to hold energy and hope again. This is not a sign that the one who has died is losing his or her place in your heart and mind. It is a sign that you are still alive and able to reinvent your life without that person. Awareness of your ability to go on can bring peace and a sense of renewal. It also affirms that while your journey as a spiritual companion to the one who died was important and will shape who you are from here on, it is now ended, and you have come home to live again.